DISEASE PREVENTION STRATEGIES

A Comprehensive Guide to Lifelong Health

By Nathan Tyler

Table of contents

Introduction

Why Prevention Matters

Prevention is the cornerstone of living a long, healthy, and fulfilling life. While modern medicine has made incredible strides in treating illnesses, the best cure remains the one you never need. Chronic diseases like heart disease, diabetes, and cancer account for the majority of global deaths—but many of these conditions are preventable. By adopting proactive measures, you can significantly reduce your risk of illness and enhance your quality of life.

Prevention isn't just about avoiding sickness; it's about thriving. Imagine waking up each day with energy, clarity, and a sense of purpose. By prioritizing health, you not only improve your own life but also reduce the burden on healthcare systems and your loved ones. Prevention empowers you to take control of your destiny rather than leaving it to chance.

The Science Behind Disease Prevention

What makes prevention so effective? The answer lies in the intricate relationship between our genetics, environment, and lifestyle. While you may inherit certain risks, your daily choices—what you eat, how much you move, how well you sleep, and how you manage stress—can significantly influence your health outcomes.

Scientific research underscores that lifestyle factors account for up to 80% of the risk for chronic diseases. For example, maintaining a healthy weight, avoiding smoking, and eating a balanced diet rich in fruits and vegetables can lower the risk of heart disease by more than 50%. Similarly, regular physical activity and stress management practices have been shown to improve immunity and even reduce the likelihood of certain cancers.

Modern advancements, like epigenetics, reveal that our behaviors can "turn on" or "turn off" specific genes, offering a powerful tool for preventing disease. Prevention, therefore, is not just a passive hope but an active science-driven approach to creating better health.

How to Use This Book

This book is your guide to taking charge of your health and making informed, intentional decisions. Designed for readers of all backgrounds, it breaks down complex medical concepts into simple, actionable steps. Each chapter focuses on a key aspect of prevention—nutrition, exercise, mental well-being, and more—equipping you with tools to transform your life one habit at a time.

Here's how to navigate the book effectively:

1. **Start with the Basics**: If you're new to the idea of prevention, focus on the foundational chapters covering risk factors, nutrition, and exercise.

2. **Tailor Your Journey**: Use the self-assessments and personalized plans to identify areas where you can make the biggest impact.

3. **Go Deep on Key Topics**: Interested in specific diseases? Explore the targeted chapters on heart health, diabetes, and cancer prevention.

4. **Take Action**: Each chapter ends with actionable tips, checklists, or templates to help you implement what you've learned.

5. **Revisit and Revise**: Prevention is a lifelong journey. Use this book as a reference guide, returning to chapters as your needs evolve.

By the end of this book, you'll not only understand the "why" of prevention but also the "how." Whether you're looking to safeguard your health, support loved ones, or simply live a more vibrant life, this book will empower you with the knowledge and confidence to take meaningful action.

Let's embark on this journey together—because your health is worth it.

Chapter 1: Understanding Your Risk Factors

When it comes to preventing diseases, knowledge is power. Understanding your risk factors allows you to take proactive measures to protect your health. These risk factors can be broadly categorized into three main areas: genetics, lifestyle, and environment. Each plays a crucial role in determining your overall health and disease susceptibility.

Genetics: Your Biological Blueprint

Your genetic makeup is the blueprint your body follows. It determines traits like eye color, height, and, unfortunately, susceptibility to certain diseases. Conditions such as heart disease, diabetes, and some forms of cancer often have a hereditary component. If your parents or grandparents faced these illnesses, your risk might be higher.

However, genetics is not destiny. The emerging field of **epigenetics** shows that lifestyle choices and environmental factors can influence how your genes are expressed. For example, while you may inherit a predisposition to diabetes, maintaining a healthy weight and active lifestyle can prevent those genes from activating.

Action Step: Review your family's medical history to identify potential hereditary risks. Share this information with your healthcare provider, as it can guide your prevention strategies.

Lifestyle: Choices That Shape Your Health

Lifestyle factors, unlike genetics, are entirely within your control. They include your diet, physical activity, sleep patterns, stress management, and habits such as smoking or alcohol consumption. Over time, unhealthy lifestyle choices can accumulate, increasing your risk for chronic diseases.

For example:

- A sedentary lifestyle increases the risk of obesity, heart disease, and diabetes.

- Chronic stress can weaken the immune system and contribute to high blood pressure.

- Poor dietary choices can lead to inflammation, a key driver of many chronic conditions.

The Good News: Small, consistent changes can make a significant difference. Choosing nutrient-dense foods, staying physically active, and prioritizing rest are steps you can take to dramatically reduce your risk.

Action Step: Reflect on your daily habits. Are there areas where you can make healthier choices? Start with one change—such as replacing sugary snacks with fruits—and build from there.

Environment: The World Around You

Your environment includes everything from the air you breathe to the community you live in. Exposure to pollutants, toxins, and even high levels of noise can negatively impact your health. Additionally, factors like access to healthcare, education, and safe recreational spaces play a significant role in your well-being.

For instance:

- Air pollution has been linked to respiratory and cardiovascular diseases.

- Prolonged exposure to harmful chemicals, such as pesticides or industrial toxins, can increase cancer risk.

- Living in a supportive community can enhance mental and emotional health.

Action Step: Evaluate your environment. Are there changes you can make, such as using air purifiers, consuming organic foods, or advocating for safer community spaces?

Self-Assessment: Identifying Your Vulnerabilities

Understanding your risk factors requires introspection and action. A self-assessment can help you identify vulnerabilities and prioritize areas for improvement. Use the questions below to get started:

Genetics:

- Do you have a family history of chronic diseases like diabetes, heart disease, or cancer?

- Are there hereditary conditions that your relatives have faced?

Lifestyle:

- How often do you exercise?

- Is your diet balanced and rich in whole, nutrient-dense foods?

- Do you manage stress effectively, or does it feel overwhelming?

- How much sleep do you get each night?

Environment:

- Are you exposed to pollutants, toxins, or harmful chemicals regularly?

- Do you have access to clean water, fresh food, and healthcare?

- Is your living space conducive to mental and physical health?

Next Steps:

1. **Identify Priorities**: Highlight areas where you are most at risk.

2. **Set Goals**: Choose specific, measurable goals to address each area.

3. **Seek Support**: Consult healthcare providers, join wellness programs, or connect with community resources for guidance.

By understanding the interplay between genetics, lifestyle, and environment, you empower yourself to take charge of your health. Prevention begins with awareness—knowing your vulnerabilities is the first step toward building a healthier, brighter future.

Chapter 2: The Role of Nutrition in Prevention

When it comes to disease prevention, nutrition is one of the most powerful tools at your disposal. Food is more than just fuel—it's medicine for the body, mind, and soul. Every bite you take has the potential to either promote health or contribute to disease. By understanding the role of nutrition, you can make choices that nourish your body, reduce the risk of chronic illnesses, and enhance your overall quality of life.

Superfoods for Longevity

Superfoods are nutrient-dense foods packed with vitamins, minerals, antioxidants, and other bioactive compounds that support health and longevity. While no single food is a magic cure-all, incorporating superfoods into your diet can provide powerful health benefits over time.

Top Superfoods for Disease Prevention

1. Berries

- Rich in antioxidants like anthocyanins, berries help fight free radicals and reduce inflammation.

- Studies link regular berry consumption to improved brain health and reduced risk of heart disease.

- **How to Use**: Add blueberries or strawberries to your morning oatmeal or smoothies.

2. Leafy Greens

- Spinach, kale, and Swiss chard are loaded with vitamins A, C, and K, as well as folate and fiber.

- They support heart health, lower blood pressure, and promote a healthy gut.

- **How to Use:** Sauté with garlic and olive oil or blend into a green smoothie.

3. Fatty Fish

- Salmon, mackerel, and sardines are excellent sources of omega-3 fatty acids, which reduce inflammation and support brain and heart health.

- **How to Use**: Grill or bake with herbs and serve alongside vegetables.

4. Nuts and Seeds

- Almonds, walnuts, chia seeds, and flax seeds provide healthy fats, protein, and fiber.

- They help regulate blood sugar, lower cholesterol, and support brain function.

- **How to Use**: Sprinkle on salads or eat as a snack.

5. Turmeric

- This golden spice contains curcumin, a potent anti-inflammatory compound.

- Regular consumption may reduce the risk of Alzheimer's, cancer, and arthritis.

- **How to Use**: Add to soups, stews, or golden milk lattes.

6. Legumes

- Lentils, chickpeas, and black beans are rich in protein, fiber, and essential nutrients like magnesium.

- They help stabilize blood sugar, improve digestion, and lower cholesterol.

- **How to Use**: Include them in salads, soups, or as a side dish.

The Power of Anti-Inflammatory Diets

Chronic inflammation is a silent contributor to many diseases, including heart disease, diabetes, cancer, and arthritis. An anti-inflammatory diet focuses on whole, nutrient-rich foods that combat inflammation while minimizing pro-inflammatory foods.

Key Components of an Anti-Inflammatory Diet

1. **Focus on Whole Foods**

- Prioritize fruits, vegetables, whole grains, lean proteins, and healthy fats.

- Limit processed foods, refined sugars, and artificial additives.

2. **Incorporate Healthy Fats**

- Omega-3 fatty acids, found in fish, flaxseeds, and walnuts, are particularly effective at reducing inflammation.

- Avoid trans fats and limit saturated fats.

3. **Spice It Up**

- Turmeric, ginger, garlic, and cinnamon are natural anti-inflammatory agents.

4. **Reduce Sugars and Refined Carbs**

- High sugar intake can trigger inflammation and raise your risk for obesity and diabetes.

- Opt for whole grains and natural sweeteners like honey or maple syrup in moderation.

5. **Hydrate Well**

- Staying hydrated helps flush toxins that contribute to inflammation.

- Include herbal teas and infused water for variety.

Benefits of an Anti-Inflammatory Diet

- Reduces the risk of chronic diseases.

- Supports joint health and reduces pain.

- Improves digestion and gut health.

- Promotes clearer skin and better energy levels.

Meal Plans and Recipes for Disease Prevention

Creating a meal plan focused on disease prevention ensures you get the nutrients your body needs daily. Here's an example of a simple, balanced plan:

Sample Day of Eating for Disease Prevention

Breakfast:

- Anti-inflammatory green smoothie: Spinach, banana, frozen blueberries, almond milk, chia seeds, and a dash of turmeric.

- Whole-grain toast with avocado and a sprinkle of flaxseeds.

Snack:

- A handful of mixed nuts and a small apple.

Lunch:

- Quinoa salad with mixed greens, cherry tomatoes, cucumber, chickpeas, and olive oil-lemon dressing.

- A small side of roasted sweet potatoes.

Snack:

- Carrot sticks with hummus.

Dinner:

- Grilled salmon with a side of sautéed kale and garlic.

- Steamed broccoli drizzled with tahini.

Dessert:

- Fresh berries with a dollop of plain Greek yogurt and a drizzle of honey.

Easy Recipes for Disease Prevention

1. Golden Turmeric Latte

- **Ingredients**: Unsweetened almond milk, turmeric powder, cinnamon, ginger, and a pinch of black pepper.

- **Directions**: Warm the almond milk and whisk in the spices. Sweeten with honey if desired.

2. Mediterranean Chickpea Salad

- **Ingredients**: Chickpeas, cucumber, cherry tomatoes, red onion, parsley, olive oil, and lemon juice.

- **Directions**: Toss all ingredients together and season with salt and pepper.

3. Berry Chia Pudding

- **Ingredients**: Chia seeds, almond milk, vanilla extract, and mixed berries.

- **Directions**: Combine chia seeds, milk, and vanilla. Let sit overnight and top with berries before serving.

Chapter 3: The Importance of Physical Activity

Physical activity is one of the most effective tools for maintaining health and preventing disease. Beyond helping with weight management, exercise strengthens the heart, improves circulation, boosts mental well-being, and even slows the aging process. A sedentary lifestyle, on the other hand, is a major risk factor for conditions like heart disease, diabetes, and obesity. Regular movement is essential for a healthy body, sharp mind, and resilient spirit.

Why Physical Activity Matters

1. **Disease Prevention:** Exercise lowers the risk of chronic illnesses like hypertension, type 2 diabetes, and certain cancers. It also helps regulate blood sugar and reduces inflammation.

2. **Mental Health Benefits**: Physical activity releases endorphins, the body's natural mood elevators. Regular exercise can reduce stress,

combat anxiety, and alleviate symptoms of depression.

3. **Improved Mobility and Longevity:** Maintaining strength, flexibility, and endurance helps preserve independence as you age and reduces the risk of falls.

4. **Enhanced Cognitive Function**: Studies show that regular exercise improves memory, focus, and overall brain health, lowering the risk of neurodegenerative diseases like Alzheimer's.

Exercise Guidelines for All Ages

Physical activity is beneficial at every stage of life, but the intensity, type, and duration of exercise should be tailored to individual needs and abilities. Here are general guidelines by age group:

Children and Adolescents (6–17 Years)

- **Recommended Activity:** At least 60 minutes of moderate to vigorous physical activity daily.

- **Focus**: Aerobic activities like running or cycling, strength-building activities like climbing or push-ups, and bone-strengthening exercises like jumping or skipping.

- **Benefits**: Supports growth, builds strong bones and muscles, and improves mental health and academic performance.

Adults (18–64 Years)

- **Recommended Activity**: At least 150 minutes of moderate-intensity aerobic activity or 75 minutes of vigorous activity per week, plus two days of muscle-strengthening exercises.

- **Focus**: A mix of cardio, strength training, and flexibility exercises to maintain overall fitness and prevent chronic diseases.

- **Benefits**: Helps maintain weight, reduces the risk of chronic illnesses, and boosts energy and mood.

Older Adults (65+ Years)

- **Recommended Activity**: Follow adult guidelines if possible, but include balance and flexibility exercises to reduce fall risk.

- **Focus**: Low-impact activities like walking, yoga, or swimming. Strength training can help combat age-related muscle loss.

- **Benefits**: Promotes independence, prevents mobility issues, and enhances cognitive health.

Special Considerations:

- Consult a healthcare provider before starting a new exercise routine, especially if you have pre-existing conditions.

- Adapt activities to suit individual fitness levels and physical limitations.

How to Stay Active with a Busy Schedule

Finding time for exercise can be challenging in today's fast-paced world, but with some creativity and planning, you can integrate physical activity into your daily routine.

1. Make Movement a Priority

- Schedule exercise as you would an important meeting. Block out time in your calendar and treat it as non-negotiable.

2. Incorporate Activity into Daily Tasks

- Take the stairs instead of the elevator.

- Park further away from your destination to add extra steps.

- Do stretches or light exercises while watching TV or during work breaks.

3. Embrace Short Workouts

- High-Intensity Interval Training (HIIT) can deliver great benefits in just 15–20 minutes.

- Micro-workouts (5–10 minutes) spread throughout the day can be just as effective as a single longer session.

4. Combine Social Time with Exercise

- Walk or jog with a friend.

- Join group classes or sports teams to make exercise enjoyable and social.

5. Use Technology to Stay Accountable

- Fitness apps, wearable trackers, or online classes can help you stay motivated and consistent.

6. Turn Everyday Chores into Exercise

- Gardening, cleaning, and carrying groceries can count as physical activity. Make them more vigorous to boost your fitness.

Quick Tip: The key is consistency. Even 10-minute bursts of activity add up over time.

Strength, Flexibility, and Cardio: A Balanced Approach

A comprehensive fitness routine should include three key components: strength, flexibility, and cardiovascular exercise. Together, they provide a holistic approach to health and prevent imbalances.

1. Strength Training: Build Muscle, Boost Metabolism

- **What It Is**: Activities that build muscle and increase bone density, such as weightlifting, resistance band exercises, or bodyweight workouts like squats and push-ups.

- **Benefits**:

    - Improves muscle tone and strength.

- Supports bone health, reducing the risk of osteoporosis.

- Increases metabolism, aiding in weight management.

- **Frequency**: At least two days per week, targeting major muscle groups.

2. Flexibility: Enhance Range of Motion

- **What It Is**: Activities that stretch muscles and improve joint mobility, such as yoga, Pilates, or simple stretching routines.

- **Benefits**:

  - Reduces the risk of injuries and muscle stiffness.

  - Improves posture and alignment.

  - Enhances relaxation and stress relief.

- **Frequency**: Include flexibility exercises daily or at least after each workout.

3. Cardiovascular Exercise: Strengthen Your Heart

- **What It Is**: Activities that increase your heart rate, such as walking, running, swimming, or cycling.

- **Benefits**:

    - Improves heart and lung function.

    - Aids in weight loss and calorie burning.

    - Boosts endurance and energy levels.

- **Frequency**: Aim for at least 150 minutes of moderate-intensity cardio per week.

Creating Your Balanced Routine

A balanced weekly plan might look like this:

- **Monday**: 30-minute brisk walk (cardio) + 15 minutes of stretching (flexibility).

- **Tuesday**: 20 minutes of strength training + 10 minutes of yoga.

- **Wednesday**: 30 minutes of cycling (cardio).

- **Thursday**: 15 minutes of bodyweight exercises + 15 minutes of stretching.

- **Friday**: 20-minute jog or HIIT workout (cardio).

- **Saturday**: Rest or light activity like a leisurely walk.

- **Sunday**: 30 minutes of swimming or dancing (cardio) + 10 minutes of flexibility work.

Chapter 4. Sleep: Your Body's Time to Heal

Sleep is not merely a time when the body rests; it is an active, dynamic process crucial for physical restoration, mental rejuvenation, and overall well-being. While you sleep, your body performs essential tasks such as repairing tissues, consolidating memories, regulating hormones, and strengthening the immune system. Neglecting sleep can lead to more than just daytime fatigue—it increases your risk of chronic diseases and accelerates aging.

The Connection Between Sleep and Chronic Diseases

Inadequate sleep doesn't just leave you groggy; it profoundly impacts your long-term health. Research has established strong links between poor sleep and the development of chronic illnesses.

1. Cardiovascular Diseases

- Sleep deprivation disrupts the body's ability to regulate blood pressure and heart rate, increasing the risk of hypertension, heart attacks, and strokes.

- During sleep, your heart rate and blood pressure naturally dip—a process essential for cardiovascular health. Without sufficient rest, this recovery mechanism is compromised.

2. Diabetes and Metabolic Disorders

- Poor sleep affects insulin sensitivity, making it harder for the body to regulate blood sugar levels. This can lead to type 2 diabetes over time.

- Sleep loss also disrupts appetite-regulating hormones, increasing cravings for high-calorie, sugary foods and contributing to weight gain.

3. Immune System Impairment

- During deep sleep, the body produces cytokines—proteins that help fight infection and inflammation. Chronic sleep deprivation weakens this response, making you more vulnerable to illnesses.

- Vaccinations are less effective in individuals who don't get adequate sleep, as the body's ability to produce antibodies is reduced.

4. Mental Health Issues

- Sleep and mental health are deeply intertwined. Poor sleep contributes to anxiety, depression, and mood disorders.

- Insufficient sleep affects the brain's ability to regulate emotions, leading to heightened irritability and stress.

5. Neurodegenerative Diseases

- Sleep plays a critical role in clearing out toxins, including beta-amyloid proteins linked to Alzheimer's disease.

- Chronic sleep deprivation increases the risk of cognitive decline and memory impairments.

Tips for Better Sleep Hygiene

Improving sleep quality begins with adopting good sleep hygiene practices—habits and routines that promote a restful night.

1. Establish a Consistent Sleep Schedule

- Go to bed and wake up at the same time every day, even on weekends. A regular sleep schedule helps regulate your body's internal clock.

2. Create a Relaxing Bedtime Routine

- Develop calming pre-sleep rituals, such as reading, meditating, or taking a warm bath.

- Avoid stimulating activities, like intense workouts or engaging in stressful conversations, close to bedtime.

3. Optimize Your Sleep Environment

- **Darkness**: Use blackout curtains or an eye mask to block out light, as darkness signals your body to produce melatonin, the sleep hormone.

- **Quiet**: Minimize noise with earplugs or a white noise machine.

- **Comfort**: Invest in a supportive mattress, pillows, and breathable bedding.

4. Limit Screen Time Before Bed

- The blue light emitted by phones, tablets, and computers interferes with melatonin production, making it harder to fall asleep.

- Aim to power down devices at least 1–2 hours before bedtime.

5. Watch What You Eat and Drink

- Avoid heavy meals, caffeine, and alcohol in the hours leading up to bedtime.

- While alcohol may make you feel drowsy initially, it disrupts sleep cycles and reduces overall sleep quality.

6. Get Regular Physical Activity

- Exercise promotes better sleep, but timing matters. Aim to work out earlier in the day, as late-night exercise can be too stimulating.

7. Manage Stress and Anxiety

- Practice relaxation techniques like deep breathing, progressive muscle relaxation, or mindfulness meditation.

- Journaling before bed can help you offload worries and clear your mind.

8. Limit Naps

- If you nap during the day, keep it short (20–30 minutes) and avoid napping too late, as this can interfere with nighttime sleep.

9. Keep Your Bedroom for Sleep

- Reserve your bed for sleep and intimacy only—avoid working, watching TV, or using your phone in bed. This trains your brain to associate your bed with rest.

10. Seek Professional Help if Needed

- If you experience persistent insomnia, sleep apnea, or other sleep disorders, consult a healthcare provider or sleep specialist. Treatment options, such as cognitive-behavioral therapy for insomnia (CBT-I) or continuous positive airway pressure (CPAP) for sleep apnea, can improve sleep quality.

Benefits of Prioritizing Quality Sleep

By improving your sleep habits, you can:

- Reduce the risk of chronic diseases like heart disease, diabetes, and Alzheimer's.

- Enhance mental clarity, focus, and productivity.

- Strengthen your immune system to fight off infections.

- Improve emotional resilience and mood stability.

- Increase energy levels and overall vitality.

Chapter 5: Heart Health

Heart disease remains one of the leading causes of death worldwide, yet it is largely preventable through lifestyle choices and proactive management of risk factors. Prioritizing heart health involves understanding its key components—cholesterol levels, blood pressure, and inflammation—and implementing strategies to optimize these areas. By taking action today, you can significantly reduce your risk of developing heart disease and enjoy a longer, healthier life.

Strategies to Prevent Heart Disease

Heart disease prevention starts with a commitment to a heart-friendly lifestyle. These strategies provide a roadmap for safeguarding your cardiovascular system:

1. Maintain a Balanced Diet

- Focus on whole, nutrient-dense foods that support heart health.

- **Emphasize:**

- **Fruits and Vegetables**: Rich in antioxidants, they combat oxidative stress, a major contributor to heart disease.

- **Whole Grains:** Foods like oats, quinoa, and brown rice are high in fiber, which helps lower cholesterol levels.

- **Healthy Fats:** Incorporate sources of omega-3 fatty acids, such as fatty fish, walnuts, and flaxseeds, to reduce inflammation.

- **Lean Proteins:** Choose skinless poultry, beans, and legumes over red and processed meats.

2. Stay Physically Active

- Regular exercise strengthens the heart muscle and improves circulation.

- Aim for **at least 150 minutes of moderate-intensity aerobic**

exercise per week, such as brisk walking, cycling, or swimming.

- Include strength training twice a week to maintain muscle mass and metabolic health.

3. Avoid Tobacco Products

- Smoking damages blood vessels, reduces oxygen flow, and increases the risk of atherosclerosis.

- Quitting smoking significantly improves heart health, even if you've been a smoker for years.

4. Manage Stress Effectively

- Chronic stress triggers hormonal changes that increase blood pressure and inflammation.

- Incorporate relaxation techniques such as meditation, yoga, or deep breathing exercises into your daily routine.

5. Maintain a Healthy Weight

- Excess body weight puts additional strain on the heart and is linked to higher cholesterol, blood pressure, and blood sugar levels.

- A balanced diet and regular exercise can help achieve and sustain a healthy weight.

6. Limit Alcohol Consumption

- While moderate alcohol intake may have some benefits, excessive drinking raises blood pressure and contributes to weight gain.

- Stick to recommended guidelines: one drink per day for women and two drinks per day for men.

7. Get Regular Checkups

- Routine medical exams can detect early signs of heart disease, allowing for timely intervention.

- Key screenings include blood pressure, cholesterol levels, blood sugar, and weight assessments.

Cholesterol, Blood Pressure, and Inflammation Management

1. Managing Cholesterol Levels

Cholesterol is essential for various bodily functions, but an imbalance can lead to plaque buildup in arteries, increasing the risk of heart attacks and strokes.

- **Types of Cholesterol**:

  - **LDL (Low-Density Lipoprotein):** Known as "bad" cholesterol, it contributes to arterial blockages.

  - **HDL (High-Density Lipoprotein):** Known as "good" cholesterol, it helps remove excess cholesterol from the bloodstream.

- **Strategies to Lower LDL Cholesterol:**

  - Reduce intake of saturated and trans fats found in processed foods, fried items, and full-fat dairy.

  - Increase soluble fiber consumption from foods like oats, beans, and apples to help remove cholesterol from the body.

  - Add plant sterols and stanols (found in fortified foods) to naturally lower LDL levels.

- **Boosting HDL Cholesterol:**

  - Engage in regular physical activity.

  - Incorporate healthy fats, such as olive oil and fatty fish, into your diet.

2. Controlling Blood Pressure

High blood pressure, or hypertension, forces the heart to work harder, leading to damage over time.

- **Dietary Changes:**

    - Follow the DASH (Dietary Approaches to Stop Hypertension) diet, which emphasizes fruits, vegetables, lean proteins, and low-sodium foods.

    - Limit salt intake to less than 2,300 milligrams per day (1,500 mg is ideal for those with hypertension).

- **Lifestyle Adjustments:**

    - Exercise regularly to improve vascular health.

    - Limit caffeine intake, as it can temporarily raise blood pressure.

- **Medication**:

  - If prescribed, adhere to medication regimens to keep blood pressure within a healthy range.

3. Reducing Inflammation

Chronic inflammation is a silent contributor to heart disease, often exacerbated by poor diet, stress, and sedentary behavior.

- **Dietary Approaches:**

  - Incorporate anti-inflammatory foods like berries, leafy greens, turmeric, and green tea.

  - Avoid processed foods, sugary drinks, and excess red meat.

- **Lifestyle Tips:**

  - Manage stress with mindfulness or relaxation techniques.

- Get adequate sleep, as poor sleep can heighten inflammation.

Heart-Healthy Habits for Life

Adopting these habits isn't about short-term fixes; it's about creating a lifestyle that prioritizes heart health for the long run:

- **Plan Your Meals:** Meal prep with heart-healthy recipes to reduce reliance on fast food.

- **Find an Exercise Buddy**: Staying active is easier when you have a partner for motivation.

- **Celebrate Small Wins**: Every positive change, no matter how small, contributes to a healthier heart.

Chapter 6: Diabetes Prevention

Diabetes, particularly type 2, has become a global health challenge. Despite its prevalence, it is largely preventable and manageable through proactive lifestyle changes. Understanding the factors that contribute to diabetes and adopting strategies to maintain healthy blood sugar levels can significantly reduce your risk. This chapter explores natural ways to prevent diabetes and improve insulin sensitivity, empowering you to take control of your health.

Managing Blood Sugar Levels Naturally

Blood sugar regulation is crucial for overall health. Persistent high blood sugar levels can lead to insulin resistance, a hallmark of type 2 diabetes. Managing blood sugar naturally involves adopting sustainable habits that promote balance and stability.

1. Understand the Glycemic Index (GI)

The glycemic index measures how quickly a carbohydrate-containing food raises blood sugar levels. Choosing low-GI foods helps maintain stable blood sugar.

- **Low-GI Foods**: Whole grains, legumes, non-starchy vegetables, nuts, and seeds.

- **High-GI Foods to Avoid**: Sugary snacks, white bread, white rice, and processed cereals.

2. Embrace Whole Foods Over Processed Options

- **Whole Foods:** Rich in fiber and nutrients, whole foods slow down sugar absorption, preventing spikes in blood sugar.

- **Processed Foods**: Often high in sugar and low in nutrients, they contribute to erratic blood sugar levels.

3. Prioritize Balanced Meals

Balanced meals combine carbohydrates, proteins, and healthy fats to slow digestion and stabilize blood sugar levels.

- **Carbohydrates**: Choose complex carbs like quinoa, sweet potatoes, and oats.

- **Proteins**: Incorporate lean meats, eggs, tofu, and legumes.

- **Healthy Fats:** Include avocado, olive oil, and fatty fish like salmon.

4. Stay Hydrated

Dehydration can affect blood sugar control. Drinking enough water helps kidneys eliminate excess sugar through urine.

5. Regular Physical Activity

Exercise helps muscle cells use glucose for energy, reducing blood sugar levels and improving insulin sensitivity.

- **Aerobic Exercise**: Brisk walking, cycling, or swimming for at least 150 minutes per week.

- **Strength Training**: Builds muscle mass, which helps burn glucose more efficiently.

6. Manage Stress Levels

Chronic stress triggers the release of cortisol, a hormone that increases blood sugar levels.

- Practice mindfulness, yoga, or deep breathing exercises to reduce stress.

7. Get Quality Sleep

Sleep deprivation impairs glucose metabolism and increases the risk of insulin resistance. Aim for 7–8 hours of restful sleep each night.

Diet and Lifestyle Tips for Insulin Sensitivity

Insulin sensitivity refers to how effectively the body's cells respond to insulin, the hormone responsible for transporting glucose from the bloodstream into cells. Enhancing insulin sensitivity is key to diabetes prevention.

1. Optimize Your Diet for Insulin Sensitivity

Certain foods can boost your cells' responsiveness to insulin:

- **Leafy Greens**: Spinach, kale, and Swiss chard are low in calories and carbohydrates but rich in magnesium, which supports insulin function.

- **Cinnamon**: Adding cinnamon to your diet may help reduce insulin resistance by lowering fasting blood sugar levels.

- **Apple Cider Vinegar**: Consuming a small amount before meals can improve insulin sensitivity and lower post-meal blood sugar spikes.

- **Nuts and Seeds**: Almonds, walnuts, and chia seeds provide healthy fats and nutrients that aid in blood sugar control.

2. Incorporate Intermittent Fasting

Intermittent fasting can improve insulin sensitivity by giving your body a break from constant glucose processing. Common methods include:

- **16:8 Method**: Fasting for 16 hours and eating within an 8-hour window.

- **5:2 Method**: Eating normally for five days and reducing calorie intake for two non-consecutive days.

3. Maintain a Healthy Weight

Excess body fat, especially around the abdomen, contributes to insulin resistance. Losing even 5–10% of your body weight can significantly improve insulin sensitivity.

4. Avoid Sedentary Behavior

Prolonged sitting or inactivity can worsen insulin resistance. Take regular breaks to move, even if it's just standing up and stretching for a few minutes every hour.

5. Limit Sugar and Refined Carbohydrates

High sugar consumption leads to rapid blood sugar spikes, taxing your body's ability to produce insulin effectively. Choose natural sweeteners like stevia or monk fruit instead.

6. Include Probiotics in Your Diet

Gut health plays a crucial role in insulin sensitivity. Probiotic-rich foods like yogurt, kefir, and fermented vegetables help maintain a healthy gut microbiome, which supports glucose metabolism.

7. Supplement Wisely

Certain supplements may enhance insulin sensitivity and prevent blood sugar spikes:

- **Magnesium**: Found in foods like nuts, seeds, and leafy greens, magnesium supports glucose metabolism.

- **Chromium**: May help improve insulin sensitivity, but consult a healthcare provider before supplementing.

- **Omega-3 Fatty Acids**: Found in fish oil, they reduce inflammation and improve insulin function.

Tracking Progress and Staying Motivated

Consistency is key when it comes to managing blood sugar and improving insulin sensitivity. Use these tips to stay on track:

- **Keep a Food Diary**: Track meals to identify patterns and make informed adjustments.

- **Monitor Blood Sugar Levels**: Use a glucometer to measure fasting and post-meal blood sugar levels regularly.

- **Celebrate Small Wins**: Acknowledge progress, whether it's weight loss, improved energy levels, or better blood sugar readings.

Chapter 7: Cancer Prevention

Cancer is a complex group of diseases characterized by uncontrolled cell growth and spread to other parts of the body. It remains one of the leading causes of death globally, but the good news is that many cancers are preventable through lifestyle choices and early detection. By understanding the factors that contribute to cancer development and adopting habits that reduce your risk, you can take significant steps toward protecting your health. This section delves into the foods, habits, and screening strategies that play a critical role in cancer prevention.

Foods and Habits That Lower Cancer Risk

Diet and lifestyle choices are integral to cancer prevention. Many factors, including oxidative stress, inflammation, and DNA damage, contribute to cancer development. Certain foods and habits can help protect your cells and reduce your risk of developing cancer.

1. Antioxidant-Rich Foods

Antioxidants protect cells from oxidative stress, which can cause DNA damage and lead to cancer. Including antioxidant-rich foods in your diet can help neutralize free radicals and prevent cellular damage.

- **Fruits and Vegetables**: Berries, citrus fruits, leafy greens, and cruciferous vegetables (like broccoli, kale, and Brussels sprouts) are all high in antioxidants.

- **Colorful Foods**: The brighter the color, the higher the antioxidant content. Carrots, sweet potatoes, and bell peppers provide carotenoids, another powerful antioxidant group.

2. Cruciferous Vegetables

Cruciferous vegetables contain compounds like sulforaphane that help detoxify carcinogens and prevent the growth of cancer cells.

- **Examples**: Broccoli, cauliflower, cabbage, Brussels sprouts, and kale.

- These vegetables are also high in fiber, which aids in digestion and supports a healthy gut, further reducing cancer risk.

3. Whole Grains and Fiber

A diet rich in fiber has been linked to a lower risk of several types of cancer, including colorectal cancer. Fiber helps regulate blood sugar levels and promotes a healthy digestive system, both of which are critical in reducing cancer risk.

- **Whole Grains**: Oats, quinoa, brown rice, and whole wheat are excellent sources of fiber.

- **Legumes and Beans**: High in both fiber and protein, these foods help maintain a healthy weight and gut microbiome, reducing the risk of cancer.

4. Healthy Fats

Incorporating healthy fats, especially omega-3 fatty acids, is essential for cancer prevention. These fats help reduce inflammation in the body, which is linked to cancer development.

- **Sources of Omega-3s:** Fatty fish (salmon, mackerel, sardines), flaxseeds, chia seeds, and walnuts.

- **Avoid Trans Fats and Excessive Saturated Fats:** These fats, found in processed foods and certain oils, have been linked to increased cancer risk.

5. Limit Red and Processed Meat

Studies have shown that high consumption of red and processed meats can increase the risk of colorectal and other cancers.

- Opt for plant-based proteins, such as beans, lentils, and tofu, as well as lean poultry or fish as alternatives.

- If you choose to eat red meat, limit intake to a few times per week and avoid processed meats like sausages, bacon, and hot dogs.

6. Green Tea and Herbal Teas

Green tea contains catechins, potent antioxidants that may help protect cells from damage and reduce the risk of certain cancers, including breast, ovarian, and prostate cancer.

- **Herbal Teas**: Ginger, turmeric, and peppermint teas also have anti-inflammatory and antioxidant properties that may support cancer prevention.

7. Limit Alcohol Intake

Excessive alcohol consumption has been linked to an increased risk of several cancers, including breast, liver, and colorectal cancers.

- **Guidelines for Alcohol Consumption**: Women should limit their intake to one drink per day, and men to two drinks per day.

- Opt for non-alcoholic beverages like water, herbal teas, or fresh fruit juices.

8. Avoiding Overeating and Maintaining a Healthy Weight

Obesity is a significant risk factor for many types of cancer, including breast, colorectal, and pancreatic cancer. Maintaining a healthy weight through a balanced diet and regular exercise can lower your cancer risk.

The Role of Early Screening

Early detection is crucial in preventing cancer from spreading or becoming harder to treat. Regular screening tests can help identify cancer in its earliest stages, when it is more treatable and manageable. The following screening tests are recommended based on age, gender, and family history.

1. Mammograms for Breast Cancer

Mammograms are X-ray images of the breast that can detect lumps or abnormalities that may indicate breast cancer.

- **Recommendation**: Women should begin mammography screenings at age 40 and continue annually or biennially, depending on their risk factors.

- Women with a family history of breast cancer may need to start screenings earlier or undergo additional imaging like ultrasounds or MRIs.

2. Pap Smears and HPV Testing for Cervical Cancer

A Pap smear is a screening test that checks for abnormal cells in the cervix that may lead to cervical cancer.

- **Recommendation**: Women should begin Pap smear screenings at age 21, with subsequent screenings every three years. At age 30, Pap smears combined with human papillomavirus (HPV) testing are recommended every five years.

- Women who have had a hysterectomy may not need screening unless they have a history of cervical cancer or precancerous conditions.

3. Colonoscopy for Colorectal Cancer

A colonoscopy involves a camera that is inserted into the colon to check for signs of cancer or precancerous growths (polyps).

- **Recommendation**: Individuals should begin regular colonoscopies at age 45, or earlier if they have a family history of colorectal cancer or certain genetic conditions.

- If no abnormalities are found, colonoscopies may be recommended every 10 years.

4. Skin Checks for Skin Cancer

Regular self-exams and professional skin checks help detect early signs of skin cancer, particularly melanoma.

- **Recommendation**: Perform monthly self-exams to look for new moles or changes in existing moles, such as asymmetry, irregular borders, or color changes.

- A dermatologist should perform a full-body skin exam every year, especially for individuals with a history of sunburns or family history of skin cancer.

5. Prostate-Specific Antigen (PSA) Test for Prostate Cancer

The PSA test measures the level of prostate-specific antigen in the blood, which may indicate prostate cancer.

- **Recommendation**: Men should discuss the pros and cons of PSA testing with their doctor starting at age 50, or earlier if they have a family history of prostate cancer.

6. Lung Cancer Screening

Lung cancer screening is typically done with a low-dose CT scan, which is recommended for individuals at high risk due to smoking or exposure to certain environmental factors.

- **Recommendation**: Current or former smokers who are 50–80 years old and have a 20-pack-year smoking history (equivalent to smoking one pack per day for 20 years) should discuss screening with their healthcare provider.

Chapter 8: Strengthening Your Immune System

A strong immune system is your body's first line of defense against illness, infections, and chronic diseases. It helps fight off harmful invaders like bacteria, viruses, and fungi, while also maintaining balance within your body. However, a weakened immune system can make you more susceptible to illness and longer recovery times. Fortunately, there are numerous ways to enhance your immune function and reduce infection risks. This section explores strategies to boost immune health, reduce infection risks, and highlights the crucial connection between your gut and immune system.

How to Reduce Infection Risks

Infections can range from mild illnesses like the common cold to more serious conditions like pneumonia or viral infections. While exposure to pathogens is inevitable, you can take steps to minimize your risk of getting sick and improve your body's ability to ward off infections.

1. Maintain Good Hygiene Practices

Hygiene is one of the most effective ways to reduce the risk of infections. Simple practices can prevent the spread of harmful bacteria and viruses:

- **Handwashing**: Wash your hands regularly with soap and water for at least 20 seconds, especially after using the restroom, handling food, or being in public places.

- **Sanitization**: If soap and water are unavailable, use hand sanitizers containing at least 60% alcohol to kill germs.

- **Avoid Touching Your Face:** Viruses can enter your body through your eyes, nose, or mouth, so avoid touching your face with unwashed hands.

2. Stay Up-to-Date on Vaccinations

Vaccinations are vital in preventing infections from viruses like influenza, hepatitis, and COVID-19. They prepare your immune system to fight off specific pathogens before they can make you sick.

- **Routine Vaccines**: Ensure that you are up-to-date on vaccines for illnesses like the flu, tetanus, and pneumonia.

- **Targeted Vaccines**: For individuals at higher risk (e.g., elderly or immunocompromised), vaccines like the shingles vaccine or a COVID-19 booster may be recommended.

3. Strengthen Your Physical Barriers

Your body's physical barriers (skin, mucous membranes) are the first lines of defense against pathogens. Protecting these barriers enhances your ability to fend off infections.

- **Hydration**: Staying hydrated keeps your mucous membranes moist, improving their ability to trap and flush out harmful pathogens.

- **Skin Health**: A healthy skin barrier prevents bacteria and viruses from entering your body. Moisturize dry skin and avoid harsh chemicals that can compromise your skin's integrity.

4. Manage Stress

Chronic stress has been shown to weaken the immune system, making you more vulnerable to infections. Stress hormones like cortisol can suppress the effectiveness of immune responses, impairing the body's ability to fight off pathogens.

- **Stress Reduction Techniques**: Regular practice of mindfulness, meditation, yoga, or deep breathing exercises can lower stress and promote immune health.

- **Adequate Rest**: Sleep plays a critical role in immune function. Aim for 7-9 hours of quality sleep each night to enhance your body's natural defense mechanisms.

5. Exercise Regularly

Moderate, regular physical activity strengthens the immune system by improving circulation, reducing inflammation, and enhancing the function of immune cells.

- **Types of Exercise**: Aerobic activities like walking, jogging, swimming, and cycling, as well as strength training, can boost immune responses.

- **Balance**: While exercise is beneficial, excessive intense exercise can temporarily suppress immune function, so it's important to find a balance.

6. Optimize Your Diet

What you eat plays a significant role in supporting your immune system. Nutrient-dense foods provide the vitamins, minerals, and antioxidants necessary for immune function.

- **Vitamin C:** Found in citrus fruits, strawberries, bell peppers, and broccoli, vitamin C supports immune cell function and helps fight off infections.

- **Vitamin D**: Vitamin D helps regulate the immune response. Sunlight exposure, fortified foods, and supplements can boost vitamin D levels.

- **Zinc**: Zinc is essential for immune cell development and function. Sources include shellfish, meat, seeds, and legumes.

- **Probiotics**: Probiotic-rich foods like yogurt, kefir, and fermented vegetables support gut health and overall immune function.

7. Avoid Smoking and Excessive Alcohol

Both smoking and excessive alcohol consumption weaken the immune system, impairing the body's ability to fight infections.

- **Quit Smoking**: Smoking damages the respiratory system, making it easier for viruses and bacteria to enter the body.

- **Limit Alcohol Intake:** Drinking excessive amounts of alcohol can suppress immune cell activity and disrupt the gut microbiome.

The Gut-Immune System Connection

Did you know that approximately 70% of your immune system is housed in your gut? The gut plays an essential role in regulating immune responses, detecting pathogens, and protecting the body from harmful invaders. This section will explore how the health of your gut directly impacts the strength of your immune system.

1. Gut Microbiome: The Immune System's Ally

The gut microbiome refers to the trillions of bacteria, viruses, fungi, and other microorganisms that reside in your digestive tract. These microorganisms have a profound impact on immune health.

- **Beneficial Bacteria**: A diverse gut microbiome rich in beneficial bacteria promotes a balanced immune response. These good bacteria help to educate and strengthen immune cells, keeping harmful bacteria in check.

- **Dysbiosis**: An imbalance in the gut microbiome (dysbiosis) can weaken the immune system and lead to chronic inflammation, increasing the risk of autoimmune diseases, allergies, and infections.

2. The Role of Fiber in Gut Health

Fiber acts as food for beneficial gut bacteria, helping them grow and thrive. These healthy bacteria produce short-chain fatty acids (SCFAs) that have anti-inflammatory properties and promote immune function.

- **Soluble Fiber**: Found in oats, beans, lentils, and fruits, soluble fiber helps maintain a healthy gut microbiome and supports immune system function.

- **Insoluble Fiber**: Found in whole grains and vegetables, insoluble fiber aids in digestion and helps prevent gut-related issues like constipation, which can disrupt immune health.

3. Probiotics and Prebiotics for Immune Function

Probiotics are live beneficial bacteria that can be taken through fermented foods or supplements, while prebiotics are non-digestible fibers that feed these good bacteria. Together, they form a synergistic relationship to support immune health.

- **Probiotic-Rich Foods**: Yogurt, kefir, kimchi, sauerkraut, and kombucha are excellent sources of probiotics.

- **Prebiotic-Rich Foods**: Garlic, onions, asparagus, bananas, and apples are rich in prebiotics, helping nourish and grow beneficial bacteria.

4. Gut Permeability and Immune Activation

Leaky gut syndrome, a condition in which the lining of the gut becomes damaged, can lead to the leakage of toxins and undigested food particles into the bloodstream, triggering immune activation and chronic inflammation.

- **Support Gut Health**: Eating an anti-inflammatory diet, managing stress, and avoiding excessive alcohol or processed foods can help maintain the integrity of the gut lining and prevent leaky gut.

5. The Impact of Antibiotics on Gut Health

While antibiotics are essential for fighting bacterial infections, they can also disrupt the balance of the gut microbiome by killing beneficial bacteria.

- **Probiotic Supplements**: After taking antibiotics, consider taking probiotics to restore the balance of gut bacteria. Consult a healthcare provider for personalized guidance.

Chapter 9: Managing Stress for a Healthier Life

Stress is a natural part of life, but when it becomes chronic, it can take a toll on both your physical and mental well-being. From busy work schedules to personal challenges, stress triggers a cascade of chemical reactions in the body, which, if not managed properly, can contribute to a wide range of diseases. Fortunately, stress management is a skill that can be developed, and learning how to handle stress effectively can not only improve your health but also enhance your overall quality of life. In this section, we will delve into the science of stress, its effects on health, and explore practical relaxation techniques that can help restore balance in your life.

Stress and Disease: What You Need to Know

When stress is experienced in short bursts, it can actually be beneficial, sharpening focus and improving performance. However, prolonged exposure to stress—particularly chronic stress—can negatively impact nearly every system in the body, increasing the risk of developing a variety of physical and mental health problems.

1. The Stress Response: Fight or Flight

The body's natural stress response is designed to protect you in times of danger. This "fight or flight" reaction triggers the release of hormones like cortisol and adrenaline, which prepare the body to respond to immediate threats. The heart rate increases, blood flow is redirected to essential muscles, and the body becomes more alert.

However, when stress becomes chronic, this fight or flight response is activated repeatedly and without the opportunity for recovery. Over time, this can lead to a number of negative effects, such as:

- **Weakened Immune System**: Chronic stress suppresses immune function, making you more susceptible to infections, illnesses, and autoimmune diseases.

- **Cardiovascular Issues**: Prolonged stress increases heart rate and blood pressure, raising the risk of hypertension, heart disease, and stroke.

- **Digestive Problems**: Stress can interfere with digestion, leading to symptoms like bloating, constipation, diarrhea, and even conditions like irritable bowel syndrome (IBS).

- **Mental Health Issues**: Chronic stress is closely linked to anxiety, depression, and other mental health conditions. It can disrupt sleep, affect mood, and lower overall cognitive function.

- **Inflammation**: Ongoing stress can increase the production of inflammatory markers in the body, contributing to conditions like arthritis, diabetes, and autoimmune disorders.

2. The Link Between Stress and Chronic Diseases

Long-term stress is often a silent contributor to chronic diseases. It can exacerbate existing conditions or create new health issues over time. For instance:

- **Heart Disease**: The constant release of stress hormones can contribute to atherosclerosis (plaque buildup in arteries), increasing the risk of heart attacks and strokes.

- **Obesity**: Stress-induced hormonal imbalances can lead to overeating, cravings for unhealthy foods, and an increase in belly fat, which is particularly linked to higher risks of type 2 diabetes and cardiovascular disease.

- **Diabetes**: Chronic stress can raise blood sugar levels, reducing insulin sensitivity and potentially leading to the development of type 2 diabetes over time.

- **Mental Decline**: Persistent stress has been shown to shrink the hippocampus, the area of the brain responsible for memory and learning, which may contribute to cognitive decline and increase the risk of dementia.

Given the profound impact that stress has on overall health, learning how to manage stress effectively is crucial in disease prevention.

Relaxation Techniques That Work

Fortunately, there are many evidence-based relaxation techniques that can help reduce stress, restore balance, and improve both physical and mental health. The key is finding what works best for you and incorporating it regularly into your routine.

1. Deep Breathing

Deep breathing is one of the simplest and most effective stress-relief techniques. By focusing on slow, deep breaths, you activate the body's parasympathetic nervous system (the "rest and digest" system), which helps counteract the fight or flight response.

- **How to Practice Deep Breathing:**

  - Sit or lie down in a comfortable position.

- Close your eyes and take a slow, deep breath in through your nose for a count of four.

- Hold your breath for a count of four.

- Exhale slowly through your mouth for a count of six or eight.

- Repeat for several minutes, focusing on the sensation of the breath.

Deep breathing can be done anywhere and at any time—whether you're feeling stressed at work, in traffic, or before bedtime. This simple technique is an effective way to calm your nervous system and promote relaxation.

2. Meditation and Mindfulness

Meditation and mindfulness practices help train the mind to focus on the present moment, which reduces rumination and helps break the cycle of stress. By consistently practicing mindfulness, you can rewire your brain to respond more calmly to stressors.

- **How to Practice Meditation:**

- Find a quiet space and sit in a comfortable position.

- Focus on your breathing or a specific mantra (a word or phrase you repeat to yourself).

- Allow any thoughts or distractions to come and go without judgment, gently guiding your attention back to your breath or mantra.

- Start with a few minutes a day and gradually increase the time.

- **Mindfulness in Daily Life:**
Mindfulness can also be practiced informally throughout the day. This involves bringing your full attention to the present moment during routine activities, such as eating, walking, or washing dishes. This helps reduce anxiety about the past or future, focusing instead on the here and now.

3. Progressive Muscle Relaxation (PMR)

Progressive Muscle Relaxation involves systematically tensing and relaxing different muscle groups in the body. This technique helps release physical tension and promotes a sense of deep relaxation.

- **How to Practice PMR:**

    - Find a quiet place to sit or lie down.

    - Start at your feet and work your way up through your body, tensing each muscle group for about 5 seconds and then releasing for 20-30 seconds.

    - Focus on the feeling of relaxation that follows the release of tension.

    - Pay special attention to areas where you tend to hold stress, such as the shoulders, neck, and jaw.

PMR is particularly useful for reducing physical symptoms of stress, such as muscle tightness and headaches, and can be a great addition to your daily relaxation routine.

4. Yoga and Tai Chi

Both yoga and Tai Chi are gentle, low-impact exercises that combine physical movement, breathing, and mindfulness to reduce stress. These practices improve flexibility, balance, and strength while also promoting relaxation.

- Yoga:

Yoga incorporates various poses and stretches along with focused breathing techniques, making it a powerful tool for managing stress. It encourages mindfulness and helps activate the body's parasympathetic nervous system.

- Tai Chi:

Tai Chi is a Chinese martial art that involves slow, deliberate movements and deep breathing. It's often referred to as "meditation in motion," as it promotes relaxation, enhances body awareness, and reduces stress.

Both practices are ideal for people of all fitness levels and can be easily integrated into daily life.

5. Visualization and Guided Imagery

Visualization, or guided imagery, is a relaxation technique that involves imagining a peaceful, serene environment, such as a beach, forest, or meadow. By engaging your senses and fully immersing yourself in the imagery, you can induce a state of calm.

- **How to Practice Visualization:**

    - Find a quiet place and sit or lie down comfortably.

    - Close your eyes and imagine a place that makes you feel calm and relaxed.

    - Focus on the sights, sounds, and smells of this place, as if you are actually there.

    - Allow yourself to experience the peaceful feelings associated with this environment.

Guided imagery can be particularly useful in times of acute stress and can be practiced for just a few minutes to help reset your mind and body.

Chapter 10: Social and Emotional Well-Being

Human beings are inherently social creatures. Our connections with others—family, friends, coworkers, and communities—are crucial for both our emotional and physical health. In today's fast-paced, digital world, it's easy to overlook the profound impact that social interactions and emotional well-being have on disease prevention. From reducing the risk of chronic illnesses to boosting mental health, the quality of our relationships and our emotional resilience play a significant role in how we feel and how our bodies function.

In this section, we will explore the connection between social and emotional well-being and overall health. We will also look at the detrimental effects of loneliness and isolation, and how cultivating meaningful relationships can enhance both your mental and physical health.

The Link Between Loneliness and Illness

Loneliness is more than just a feeling—it is a state of mind that can have a significant impact on your health. Research has shown that chronic loneliness and social isolation can increase the risk of developing a variety of health problems, both physical and mental.

1. The Physiological Effects of Loneliness

When we feel lonely, the body experiences heightened levels of stress, including an increase in cortisol, the body's primary stress hormone. Chronic stress from loneliness can affect various systems in the body, including:

- **Immune System Weakness**: Loneliness can suppress the immune system, making it more difficult for the body to fight infections and illnesses. Studies have shown that lonely individuals are more susceptible to colds, flu, and other viral infections.

- **Inflammation**: Loneliness has been linked to higher levels of inflammation in the body, which is a contributing factor to many chronic diseases, including heart disease, diabetes, and arthritis.

- **Increased Risk of Cardiovascular Disease**: Social isolation has been shown to increase blood pressure and promote other cardiovascular risk factors, including high cholesterol and a sedentary lifestyle. Lonely individuals are at a higher risk of developing heart disease and stroke.

- **Increased Mortality Risk:** Studies indicate that loneliness can increase the risk of premature death. Some studies suggest that the negative health effects of loneliness are as harmful as smoking or obesity.

2. The Impact of Loneliness on Mental Health

Loneliness also takes a toll on mental health, contributing to feelings of depression, anxiety, and stress. The lack of social support can exacerbate these feelings, creating a vicious cycle of isolation and poor mental health.

- **Depression**: Lonely individuals are at an increased risk of developing depression. Lack of social interaction and emotional support can lead to feelings of hopelessness and worthlessness.

- **Anxiety**: Chronic loneliness can heighten feelings of anxiety, especially in social situations. People who feel disconnected may develop social anxiety or fear rejection, which only perpetuates their isolation.

- **Cognitive Decline:** Prolonged loneliness has been linked to an increased risk of cognitive decline and dementia, particularly in older adults. The lack of mental stimulation from social interaction may lead to brain atrophy, affecting memory, reasoning, and decision making skills.

Building Supportive Relationships

While loneliness can have severe health consequences, the opposite—building and maintaining supportive relationships—can significantly improve your health and quality of life. Positive social connections can help reduce stress, enhance emotional resilience, and even improve your longevity. But how can you foster these relationships and ensure that your social interactions are beneficial?

1. The Power of Social Support

Social support is one of the most important factors for emotional well-being. Having a network of people you can rely on—whether it's family, friends, or even colleagues—can buffer against the effects of stress, help you navigate difficult times, and promote a sense of belonging. The emotional support you receive from others can act as a protective factor for your mental health.

- **Reducing Stress**: Talking to a friend or loved one about your challenges can reduce feelings of stress and anxiety. Emotional support can help you gain perspective on issues and provide comfort during difficult moments.

- **Improved Coping Skills**: Supportive relationships improve your ability to cope with life's challenges. When you face adversity, having people who understand and encourage you can help you navigate tough situations more effectively.

- **Positive Impact on Physical Health**: Studies show that having strong social relationships is linked to better physical health outcomes, such as lower blood pressure, reduced inflammation, and improved immune function. People with strong social ties tend to recover more quickly from illness and live longer, healthier lives.

2. Creating Meaningful Connections

Not all social interactions are created equal. The quality of your relationships is more important than the quantity. Meaningful connections—those based on trust, empathy, and mutual support—are the ones that contribute most to your well-being.

- **Building Trust**: Trust is the foundation of any strong relationship. Be reliable, consistent, and open in your communication with others. Building trust allows you to form deeper emotional bonds that offer genuine support.

- **Empathy and Listening**: One of the most powerful ways to nurture relationships is through empathy and active listening. Show understanding and compassion toward others, and allow them to express themselves without judgment. A genuine listening ear can make all the difference in strengthening relationships.

- **Be Present**: Sometimes, the best way to build meaningful connections is to simply be present. Spend time with those you care about, whether through face-to-face interactions or virtual connections. Quality time together fosters a sense of connection and belonging.

3. Nurturing Relationships with Family and Friends

While it's important to foster new relationships, maintaining strong bonds with family and old friends is equally important. These relationships have stood the test of time,

and they often provide the deepest emotional
support.

- **Communication is Key:** Regular, open communication is essential for maintaining strong relationships. Take time to check in with loved ones, whether it's through phone calls, texts, or in-person visits.

- **Shared Activities**: Engaging in shared activities—whether it's a hobby, a family tradition, or simply spending time together—helps create lasting memories and strengthen the emotional bond between you and others.

- **Support Through Difficult Times**: During times of loss, illness, or personal challenges, leaning on family and friends can provide the emotional support you need to heal and recover.

4. Expanding Your Social Circle

If your social circle is small, it's never too late to expand it. Engaging in new activities, joining clubs, or participating in community events can open doors to new friendships and provide opportunities for personal growth.

- **Volunteer Work**: Volunteering is a great way to connect with others who share your values. Giving back to the community not only helps those in need but also fosters a sense of purpose and belonging.

- **Professional Networking**: Building relationships within your professional circle can provide support in both career and personal matters. It's essential to nurture these relationships, whether through mentorship, collaboration, or simply showing appreciation for your colleagues.

- **Engage in Hobbies and Interests**: Join clubs or groups that align with your passions and interests. Shared activities create natural opportunities to meet like-minded people and form connections.

5. Emotional Resilience and Self-Care

In addition to external relationships, it's important to nurture your emotional well-being internally. Building emotional resilience helps you better cope with life's ups and downs and reduces your vulnerability to stress.

- **Self-Compassion**: Treat yourself with the same kindness and understanding that you would offer to a friend. Self-compassion helps build emotional strength and reduces negative self-judgment.

- **Mindfulness and Emotional Awareness**: Practice mindfulness to become more aware of your emotions and how they affect your physical health. Understanding and managing your emotional responses can help you build resilience in the face of adversity.

- **Seeking Professional Support**: If you find it difficult to manage stress, anxiety, or depression on your own, seeking professional help from a therapist or counselor can be an important step toward improving your emotional well-being.

Chapter 11: The Mind-Body Connection

The mind and body are intricately connected, and understanding how this connection works can be one of the most powerful tools in disease prevention. While we often think of the body as separate from the mind, the two are deeply intertwined. Mental and emotional states can directly impact physical health, and vice versa. Chronic stress, for example, can weaken the immune system, increase inflammation, and contribute to conditions like heart disease, diabetes, and autoimmune disorders. Conversely, maintaining a healthy mind can boost physical health, improve immune function, and enhance overall well-being.

In this section, we'll explore the profound connection between the mind and body, the benefits of mindfulness and meditation for disease prevention, and mental health strategies you can incorporate into your daily routine for a healthier, more balanced life.

The Role of Mindfulness and Meditation in Prevention

Mindfulness and meditation are practices that have been around for centuries, but in recent years, they have gained widespread recognition for their profound impact on health. These practices promote relaxation, increase self-awareness, and improve emotional regulation, all of which contribute to better physical and mental health.

1. Understanding Mindfulness

Mindfulness is the practice of paying attention to the present moment without judgment. It involves observing your thoughts, emotions, and bodily sensations in a non-reactive way, allowing you to become more aware of how your body responds to stress and other stimuli. Mindfulness has been shown to have numerous benefits for both mental and physical health:

- **Stress Reduction**: Mindfulness can help lower stress levels by teaching you how to respond to challenges in a calm and composed manner, rather than reacting impulsively or negatively.

- **Improved Immune Function**: Studies have shown that mindfulness can enhance immune system activity, helping the body fight off infections more effectively.

- **Lower Blood Pressure**: Regular mindfulness practice has been associated with a reduction in blood pressure, which is crucial for heart health and overall well-being.

- **Reduced Inflammation**: Mindfulness has been found to lower markers of inflammation in the body, which plays a central role in the development of chronic diseases.

2. The Power of Meditation for Disease Prevention

Meditation is a mental exercise that involves focusing the mind and calming the body. It can take many forms, such as focusing on the breath, repeating a mantra, or visualizing peaceful imagery. Meditation has been shown to reduce the risk of many health conditions, such as:

- **Heart Disease**: Meditation has been linked to lower levels of stress, reduced blood pressure, and improved heart rate variability, all of which contribute to better cardiovascular health.

- **Anxiety and Depression**: Meditation has a powerful effect on reducing symptoms of anxiety and depression. Regular practice can help you develop a more balanced emotional state and improve overall mental health.

- **Pain Management:** Meditation has been shown to increase pain tolerance and reduce chronic pain, providing a natural way to manage pain without relying on medication.

- **Better Sleep:** Regular meditation practice promotes better sleep quality, helping you get the restorative rest your body needs for recovery and healing.

3. Incorporating Mindfulness and Meditation into Daily Life

The beauty of mindfulness and meditation lies in their simplicity and accessibility. You don't need to be in a quiet, isolated setting or have hours of free time to experience the benefits. Here are a few ways to incorporate these practices into your daily routine:

- **Mindful Breathing:** Start by taking a few moments each day to focus on your breath. Breathe in deeply through your nose, hold for a few seconds, and then exhale slowly. This simple practice can help calm your nervous system and reduce stress.

- **Body Scan Meditation**: This practice involves focusing on different parts of your body, noticing any tension or discomfort. It's a great way to reconnect with your body and release physical stress.

- **Mindful Walking**: You can practice mindfulness while walking by focusing on the sensation of your feet touching the ground, the sounds around you, and the rhythm of your breath.

- **Guided Meditation**: If you're new to meditation, using a guided meditation app or video can help you get started.

These resources can provide structure and guidance as you learn to meditate.

Mental Health Strategies for a Healthier You

While mindfulness and meditation are powerful tools for improving mental health, there are many other strategies you can adopt to promote emotional well-being and prevent mental health issues from arising.

1. Stress Management

Chronic stress is one of the leading causes of many physical and mental health problems. Learning how to manage stress is crucial for disease prevention. Here are some effective strategies for reducing stress:

- **Exercise**: Physical activity is one of the best ways to combat stress. Exercise releases endorphins, the body's natural "feel-good" chemicals, which can help lift your mood and reduce anxiety.

- **Time Management**: Poor time management can lead to stress and overwhelm. By organizing your tasks and prioritizing your responsibilities, you can reduce feelings of pressure and maintain a sense of control over your life.

- **Relaxation Techniques**: Techniques such as progressive muscle relaxation, deep breathing, or visualization can help activate the body's relaxation response, lowering heart rate and blood pressure.

- **Hobbies and Interests**: Engaging in activities you enjoy can help take your mind off stressors and provide an outlet for creativity and relaxation. Whether it's reading, painting, gardening, or playing a musical instrument, finding time for hobbies is essential for stress relief.

2. Building Emotional Resilience

Emotional resilience refers to your ability to bounce back from adversity and cope with difficult emotions. Building emotional resilience can protect your mental and physical health in the face of challenges. Here's how to strengthen your emotional resilience:

- **Develop a Positive Mindset**: Cultivate a positive outlook on life by focusing on the things you're grateful for. Keeping a gratitude journal or simply reflecting on positive moments each day can help shift your perspective.

- **Self-Compassion**: Be kind to yourself during tough times. Self-compassion involves treating yourself with the same care and understanding that you would offer to a friend. This practice can reduce negative self-talk and increase emotional well-being.

- **Accept What You Can't Control**: Part of building emotional resilience is accepting that there are some things in life you cannot control. Letting go of the need to control every situation can reduce stress and help you focus on what you can influence.

- **Social Support**: Having a support system of friends, family, or even a therapist can provide emotional strength during difficult times. Don't be afraid to reach out for help when you need it.

3. Developing Healthy Coping Mechanisms

Healthy coping mechanisms are essential for managing life's stresses and emotional challenges. Instead of resorting to unhealthy habits, such as overeating, alcohol use, or avoidance, try these healthier alternatives:

- **Journaling**: Writing down your thoughts and feelings can help you process emotions and gain clarity. Journaling is a safe space to express yourself without judgment.

- **Mindfulness and Breathing Exercises**: As mentioned earlier, mindfulness and deep breathing are excellent tools for staying grounded during stressful moments. These techniques can help you pause, reset, and approach challenges with a clear mind.

- **Therapy or Counseling**: Professional support from a therapist or counselor can be invaluable for learning how to cope with difficult emotions, trauma, or mental health conditions. Therapy provides a space for self-reflection and personal growth.

Chapter 12: Creating a Personalized Prevention Plan

A personalized prevention plan is a roadmap for maintaining and enhancing your health. It involves evaluating your current lifestyle, identifying areas for improvement, and outlining practical steps you can take to reduce your risk of disease. Everyone is different, and your prevention plan should reflect your specific health needs, challenges, and goals.

1. Assessing Your Current Health Status

The first step in creating a personalized prevention plan is to assess your current health status. This involves understanding where you stand in terms of your physical, mental, and emotional health. Consider the following:

- **Medical History**: Review your personal and family medical history to identify any inherited risks for certain diseases, such as heart disease, diabetes, or cancer.

- **Lifestyle Factors**: Reflect on your daily habits, including your diet, exercise routine, sleep patterns, stress levels, and social connections. These habits directly impact your health.

- **Current Health Indicators:** If available, assess current health metrics like cholesterol levels, blood pressure, body mass index (BMI), and blood sugar levels. These indicators can provide valuable insights into your health risks and guide your prevention plan.

- **Mental and Emotional Health:** Mental well-being is just as important as physical health. Take note of how you manage stress, whether you feel emotionally balanced, and if there are areas where you might benefit from additional support.

2. Identifying Your Health Goals

Once you've assessed your current health status, the next step is identifying your specific health goals. These could range from preventing chronic diseases like heart disease or diabetes to improving your mental well-being or boosting your energy levels. Some examples of health goals might include:

- **Improving cardiovascular health** by exercising regularly and eating a heart-healthy diet.

- **Managing stress** through mindfulness, relaxation techniques, or therapy.

- **Maintaining a healthy weight** by focusing on a balanced diet and regular physical activity.

- **Boosting immunity** by optimizing your nutrition and sleep habits.

Make sure your goals are specific, measurable, and achievable. For instance, instead of a vague goal like "eat healthier," set a specific target like "incorporate at least five servings of fruits and vegetables into my diet each day."

3. Creating Actionable Steps

After setting your goals, break them down into actionable steps. These should be small, manageable actions that you can incorporate into your daily routine. For example, if your goal is to improve cardiovascular health, your actionable steps might include:

- **Exercise Plan:** Start with 20-30 minutes of moderate-intensity exercise, such as walking or cycling, at least 4 times a week.

- **Dietary Changes**: Include heart-healthy foods like whole grains, lean proteins, and healthy fats in every meal. Aim to reduce your intake of processed foods and sugary beverages.

- **Sleep Hygiene**: Ensure you are getting 7-9 hours of sleep each night to support heart health and recovery.

4. Setting a Timeline and Deadlines

Setting a realistic timeline for achieving your goals is key to staying motivated and accountable. For example, if you aim to reduce your blood pressure, set a target of lowering it by 5 points over the next 6 months. Setting specific deadlines allows you to track progress and make adjustments along the way.

Setting Realistic Goals

The foundation of any successful prevention plan is the ability to set realistic, achievable goals. Without clear, attainable goals, it's easy to become overwhelmed or lose focus. To ensure your goals are effective and sustainable, follow these guidelines:

1. Use the SMART Criteria

One of the best ways to set goals is by using the SMART framework. SMART stands for:

- **Specific**: Your goal should be clear and specific. Instead of saying "I want to be healthier," say "I want to walk 10,000 steps every day."

- **Measurable**: You need a way to measure progress. For example, "I will drink 8 glasses of water per day" is measurable.

- **Achievable**: Set goals that are realistic given your current situation. Gradually increase the difficulty as you progress.

- **Relevant**: Your goals should align with your larger health vision. Choose goals that matter to you personally.

- **Time-bound**: Establish a time frame to reach your goals. This could be a week, a month, or a year, depending on the goal.

2. Break Large Goals into Smaller Steps

Large goals can feel daunting, so it's helpful to break them down into smaller, more manageable steps. For example, if your long-term goal is to lose 30 pounds, start by setting smaller, achievable goals like "lose 5 pounds in the next month" or "walk for 20 minutes every day this week."

3. Celebrate Milestones

Tracking and celebrating your progress is crucial for staying motivated. When you reach a milestone, take time to reflect on your success and reward yourself with something meaningful (but not unhealthy). For example, if you've successfully exercised 4 times a week for a month, treat yourself to a new workout outfit or a massage.

4. Stay Flexible

Life is unpredictable, and sometimes you may encounter setbacks or challenges that prevent you from reaching your goals on time. It's important to remain flexible and adjust your goals as necessary, rather than abandoning them altogether. If you miss a week of exercise, don't give up—just get back on track the following week.

Habit-Tracking Templates and Checklists

Tracking your progress is an essential part of staying on course with your prevention plan. It allows you to see how far you've come, recognize patterns, and make adjustments to ensure long-term success. Here are some tools you can use to stay organized and motivated:

1. Habit-Tracking Templates

A habit-tracking template is a simple way to keep track of the healthy habits you're incorporating into your routine. You can either create your own or use pre-made templates available in apps or printable formats. A typical habit tracker includes:

- **Days of the Week**: Each day is listed with checkboxes to mark off when a task is completed.

- **Habits or Actions**: The specific habits or actions you're focusing on, such as "drink 8 glasses of water," "exercise for 30 minutes," or "meditate for 10 minutes."

- **Progress Notes**: A section to write any notes or reflections about your experience, such as how you felt after completing a task or any challenges you faced.

2. Weekly and Monthly Checklists

In addition to habit trackers, weekly and monthly checklists can help you stay on track. These checklists provide an overview of your goals and the actions you need to take to reach them. At the beginning of each week or month, outline your key goals and the steps you need to take to achieve them. At the end of the week or month, review your progress and make adjustments as needed.

For example, a monthly checklist for improving your diet might look like this:

- Plan meals for the week

- Cook at least three meals from scratch

- Incorporate two servings of vegetables into every meal

- Limit processed foods to no more than twice a week

3. Digital Apps for Tracking

There are numerous apps available for tracking habits and goals. Some of the most popular ones include:

- **Habitica**: Turns goal-setting into a game, allowing you to earn rewards for completing tasks.

- **MyFitnessPal**: Great for tracking nutrition, calories, and exercise.

- **Headspace**: Focused on mindfulness and meditation tracking.

- **Strava**: A fitness app to track walking, running, and cycling activities.

Using these apps can help streamline the tracking process and give you real-time insights into your progress.

Chapter 13: Overcoming Barriers to Change

Making lasting changes to improve your health and prevent disease can be a challenging journey, especially when you encounter barriers that stand in the way of success. These barriers often include time constraints, lack of motivation, and financial limitations. However, with the right strategies and mindset, these obstacles can be overcome. This chapter will explore how to navigate these common challenges and find practical solutions. We'll also look at how involving your family and community can enhance your efforts and keep you on track.

Time, Motivation, and Financial Constraints

One of the most common barriers people face when trying to adopt healthier habits is the lack of time. Whether it's a busy career, family responsibilities, or other personal commitments, finding time to focus on prevention can seem impossible. Alongside time constraints, motivation and finances are often cited as major obstacles to lasting change. The good news is that there are strategies to overcome these challenges and create a sustainable health routine that fits your lifestyle.

1. Overcoming Time Constraints

Many people feel that they simply don't have enough time to prioritize their health. Between work, family, social obligations, and daily responsibilities, carving out time for exercise, meal prep, or self-care may feel overwhelming. However, it is possible to make health a priority by adjusting your mindset and organizing your schedule.

- **Prioritize Your Health**: The first step in overcoming time constraints is to recognize that your health is an essential investment. Just as you schedule work meetings, appointments, or social events, treat your health as a non-negotiable commitment. Scheduling time for exercise or meal prep should be as automatic as any other obligation.

- **Make Small Changes**: You don't need to dedicate hours a day to health improvements. Small changes can add up over time. For example, try shorter, high-intensity workouts (like 20-minute home sessions) or meal prep in batches to save time during the week. Every small change counts toward achieving long-term health goals.

- **Use Time Wisely:** Look for pockets of time throughout your day. For example, you can listen to educational podcasts or audiobooks while commuting or exercising. If you have a busy schedule, consider preparing meals for the week ahead on weekends or utilizing simple, quick recipes that require minimal preparation.

- **Automate Where Possible:** Automating healthy habits can also save time. Subscription services for healthy meal kits or grocery delivery can help ensure you have nutritious ingredients on hand, while fitness trackers can remind you to move throughout the day, reducing the mental load of planning each step.

2. Boosting Motivation

Staying motivated over the long term is another common challenge. It's easy to feel excited about making positive changes at the start, but maintaining that enthusiasm can be difficult when results don't come quickly, or obstacles arise. Building and sustaining motivation requires a combination of strategies.

- **Set Small, Achievable Goals**: Rather than focusing solely on long-term outcomes, break your goals into smaller, manageable steps. Achieving small successes, like walking 10,000 steps a day or cooking a healthy meal three times a week, can provide the motivation needed to continue progressing.

- **Track Your Progress**: Tracking your efforts provides tangible evidence of your progress, which can be incredibly motivating. Whether you use a fitness app, a journal, or a habit tracker, being able to look back and see the steps you've taken will reinforce the positive changes you've made.

- **Create a Support System**: Having a support system is essential to maintaining motivation. Surround yourself with people who encourage and hold you accountable. This could include family members, friends, or even online communities with similar health goals.

- **Focus on Why You Started**: Whenever motivation wanes, reconnect with your initial reasons for making a change. Remind yourself of the long-term benefits of prevention and how it will impact your quality of life.

3. Navigating Financial Constraints

The idea of investing in health can often be daunting, especially when there are financial limitations. Healthy eating, gym memberships, personal trainers, and supplements can all seem expensive. However, there are many ways to prioritize your health without breaking the bank.

- **Embrace Budget-Friendly Nutrition**: Healthy eating doesn't have to be expensive. Focus on affordable nutrient-dense foods like beans, lentils, whole grains, seasonal vegetables, and frozen fruits. Buy in bulk, shop for sales, and plan meals around inexpensive yet nutritious ingredients.

- **Utilize Free or Low-Cost Fitness Resources**: You don't need a gym membership or expensive equipment to stay active. Many online resources offer free workout videos, including yoga, bodyweight exercises, and cardio routines that can be done at home. Consider walking or jogging in local parks, which requires no cost at all.

- **DIY Self-Care:** There are countless ways to take care of your mental and physical health without spending money. Practice stress-relieving techniques like deep breathing, mindfulness, and meditation—many of which are free and require no special equipment.

- **Look for Discounts and Programs**: Many health-related products and services, such as fitness classes, nutrition consultations, or even health insurance, offer discounts or sliding scale pricing. Additionally, check for local community programs or public health initiatives that support wellness efforts.

Involving Your Family and Community

One of the most powerful ways to overcome barriers to change is by involving those around you. When you share your health goals and invite others to participate in your journey, you not only increase your accountability but also create a support network that can help you maintain your motivation.

1. Family Support: The Power of Shared Health Goals

Incorporating your family into your health journey can make it easier to stick with new habits. When everyone in your household is on the same page, you can create a supportive environment where health is a shared priority.

- **Healthier Family Meals**: If your goal is to eat healthier, involve your family in meal planning and cooking. This not only ensures everyone enjoys nutritious meals, but it also creates an opportunity for family bonding and teaches children valuable lessons about nutrition.

- **Exercise Together**: Encourage family fitness activities such as hiking, biking, or playing sports. Doing physical activities together strengthens relationships and makes exercise fun.

- **Support Each Other's Goals**: Encourage each family member to set personal health goals and offer support. Having a shared commitment to wellness can make the process more enjoyable and provide each person with a sense of accountability.

2. Building Community Support

A supportive community can also help you stay motivated and overcome challenges. This can be a formal group, such as a workout class or support group, or a more informal network of friends and neighbors.

- **Join Social Health Groups**: Participate in local health clubs, sports leagues, or online groups that promote disease prevention and wellness. Being part of a community with similar goals helps you stay motivated and gives you access to a wealth of knowledge and support.

- **Volunteer or Participate in Health Initiatives**: Many communities offer events like charity runs, health fairs, or wellness programs that encourage health improvement. Participating in these events can provide motivation and a sense of accomplishment.

- **Accountability Partners**: Find a friend, coworker, or neighbor with similar health goals to be your accountability partner. Whether it's checking in on each other's progress or working out together, having someone else to share the journey with can be highly motivating.

Chapter 14: When to Seek Professional Help

Taking a proactive approach to disease prevention is essential, but there may come a time when self-care and lifestyle adjustments are not enough. Knowing when to seek professional help can make a significant difference in your health outcomes. Many conditions can be prevented or managed more effectively when identified early. In this chapter, we'll explore how to recognize the warning signs that indicate it's time to seek professional medical advice and how to build a supportive relationship with your healthcare provider to ensure that your health is prioritized.

Recognizing Warning Signs

Our bodies are constantly communicating with us, but often we don't listen closely enough to pick up on the subtle cues that something may be wrong. Recognizing the warning signs of illness early on can make a world of difference in preventing more serious conditions or managing them more effectively. Understanding when symptoms warrant professional attention is an important skill in maintaining long-term health.

1. Persistent Symptoms

One of the key warning signs that it's time to see a healthcare professional is the persistence of symptoms. If you've been experiencing symptoms like:

- **Chronic fatigue**

- **Unexplained weight loss or gain**

- **Persistent pain**

- **Frequent headaches**

- **Changes in appetite or sleep patterns**

These ongoing or worsening symptoms could be signs of an underlying condition that needs medical evaluation. Even seemingly minor symptoms, if they persist for weeks or months, should not be ignored. An early visit to a doctor can help pinpoint the cause before it evolves into something more serious.

2. Sudden or Severe Symptoms

If you experience any sudden or severe symptoms, it's essential to seek professional help immediately. These may include:

- **Severe chest pain** or pressure

- **Difficulty breathing**

- **Sudden vision changes**

- **Unexplained bleeding**

- **Sudden weakness or numbness in limbs**

- **Sudden dizziness or fainting**

These symptoms could indicate an acute medical emergency, such as a heart attack, stroke, or other life-threatening condition. In these cases, getting immediate professional attention is crucial to minimize the risk of permanent damage or complications.

3. Mental Health Concerns

Mental health is just as important as physical health, and symptoms like persistent feelings of sadness, anxiety, or mood swings should not be ignored. If you find yourself experiencing any of the following, it may be time to seek help:

- **Constant feelings of hopelessness or despair**

- **Extreme changes in mood or behavior**

- **Difficulty concentrating or making decisions**

- **Withdrawing from social activities**

- **Thoughts of self-harm or suicide**

Mental health concerns are not always visible and can manifest in many ways. Seeking professional guidance, whether through a therapist, counselor, or psychiatrist, can help you navigate these challenges and prevent further distress.

4. Unexplained Symptoms with No Clear Diagnosis

Sometimes, we experience symptoms that don't have an immediate explanation. These might be vague, such as fatigue, digestive issues, or skin changes that don't seem to improve with over-the-counter remedies or lifestyle changes. When symptoms don't respond to basic treatments or when they persist over time, seeking medical advice can help uncover any underlying issues that require specific attention.

5. Risk Factors for Chronic Diseases

If you have risk factors for chronic diseases such as heart disease, diabetes, or cancer—especially if they run in your family—it's crucial to seek professional help for regular screenings, evaluations, and guidance on preventive measures. A healthcare provider can offer personalized advice based on your risk factors, lifestyle, and family history.

Building a Relationship with Your Healthcare Provider

Building a strong and trusting relationship with your healthcare provider is essential for maintaining your health and preventing disease. A good relationship ensures that you feel comfortable discussing all aspects of your health, enabling your doctor to offer the best advice, care, and support. This partnership allows for better communication, personalized care, and more effective prevention strategies.

1. Open and Honest Communication

One of the foundational elements of a good relationship with your healthcare provider is open and honest communication. It's important to share your health history, concerns, and symptoms without fear of judgment. Be as detailed as possible when describing your symptoms, lifestyle, and habits, as this information helps your provider make an accurate diagnosis and create a tailored plan for disease prevention.

- **Be prepared for your appointment**: Write down any symptoms, questions, or concerns you have in advance to ensure that you don't forget important details during the visit.

- **Discuss your lifestyle and goals**: Whether it's improving nutrition, increasing physical activity, or managing stress, sharing your health goals with your doctor can help them guide you more effectively.

2. Advocate for Your Health

While your healthcare provider is there to help guide and treat you, it's important to advocate for your own health as well. If you don't fully understand a diagnosis or treatment plan, don't hesitate to ask for clarification. If a certain treatment or medication doesn't seem to be working for you, communicate this openly. You should feel empowered to ask questions, request second opinions, or explore alternative options if necessary.

3. Regular Check-Ups and Screenings

Routine check-ups and screenings are essential for early detection and disease prevention. Make sure to schedule regular visits with your healthcare provider, even when you feel healthy. These check-ups provide an opportunity for your doctor to monitor your overall health, perform necessary screenings, and detect potential health issues before they become more serious.

- **Know the recommended screening guidelines** for your age, gender, and family history, and make sure to stay on top of vaccinations and preventive care.

- **Track your health milestones**: Keeping a record of your health screenings, lab results, and vaccinations can help you stay organized and ensure you don't miss any important check-ups.

4. Collaborate on Preventive Strategies

Building a relationship with your healthcare provider is not just about treatment when things go wrong—it's also about working together to prevent disease. Your doctor can offer advice on lifestyle changes, such as diet and exercise, that can help you reduce your risk of chronic diseases. They may also guide you through the process of setting realistic health goals and help you track your progress over time.

5. Choosing the Right Provider

Finding a healthcare provider you trust is essential to building a productive relationship. Whether it's a primary care physician, a specialist, or a mental health professional, it's important to feel comfortable with them. If you feel that your current provider doesn't align with your values or isn't offering the care you need, don't be afraid to seek out another provider who is a better fit for you.

Conclusion: Your Path to a Healthier Future

As you reach the end of this book, it's important to reflect on your journey toward better health and a future free from preventable diseases. This path is not one of perfection but of continuous improvement, self-awareness, and determination. Disease prevention is not a one-time effort—it's a lifelong commitment to making choices that support your well-being, from nutrition and physical activity to emotional health and stress management. By taking proactive steps now, you can lay the foundation for a future that's healthier, more vibrant, and more fulfilling.

Reflecting on Your Journey

The first step toward disease prevention often begins with awareness. As you reflect on the information you've learned throughout this book, think about the changes you've made in your life so far. Are there areas where you've already seen improvements? Perhaps you've adopted a healthier eating plan, committed to regular exercise, or started focusing on better sleep. Even small changes can lead to significant benefits over time.

Take a moment to celebrate the progress you've made, no matter how small. Preventive health is a journey, not a destination, and each step forward brings you closer to your goals. At the same time, it's important to recognize areas where you may still face challenges. Disease prevention isn't about being perfect, but about striving to make consistent, positive choices that improve your quality of life.

Reflecting on your journey helps reinforce the behaviors and habits you've incorporated into your life. It also allows you to recognize where you might need more support or where you can push yourself to improve further. Don't be discouraged if you haven't achieved everything you set out to do right away. Every day is a new opportunity to make healthier choices and move closer to your goals.

Staying Motivated and Consistent

One of the greatest challenges in maintaining a prevention-focused lifestyle is staying motivated and consistent over time. It's easy to start with enthusiasm, but over the long term, old habits can creep back in, and motivation can wane. The key to long-term success is developing sustainable habits that fit seamlessly into your daily life. Here are a few strategies to help you stay motivated and on track:

1. Set Realistic, Achievable Goals

The foundation of lasting motivation is setting clear, realistic goals that you can track and measure. Break down your larger health objectives into smaller, manageable steps. For example, instead of saying, "I want to be healthy," focus on achievable goals like "I will eat a plant-based meal twice a week" or "I will walk 30 minutes every day." As you accomplish each mini-goal, you'll feel a sense of accomplishment that propels you toward the next step.

2. Celebrate Your Progress

Take time to celebrate every success, no matter how small. Whether it's cooking a healthy meal, completing a workout, or improving your sleep habits, acknowledging your achievements helps reinforce positive behavior. Keep a journal of your progress or track it using an app—seeing how far you've come will help keep you motivated on the days when your commitment feels tested.

3. Find Your "Why"

One of the strongest motivators for sticking with your prevention plan is identifying the deeper reasons behind your health goals. Ask yourself why disease prevention is important to you. Whether it's to have more energy for your family, improve your mental clarity, or live longer and enjoy a better quality of life, connecting to your "why" can give you the drive to stay consistent even on tough days. Write it down and refer to it regularly for a reminder of your true motivation.

4. Build a Support System

Having a support system can make a world of difference in maintaining your health goals. Surround yourself with people who encourage and support your journey, whether it's family, friends, or a community group. You might even consider joining a health-related challenge or support group, where you can share experiences, challenges, and victories with others. Sharing your journey with others not only helps you stay accountable but also provides the encouragement you need to push through tough moments.

5. Be Kind to Yourself

Lastly, remember that setbacks are a natural part of any journey. You may slip up now and then, but that doesn't mean you've failed. Rather than feeling guilty or discouraged, take these moments as opportunities to learn and adjust your approach. Be compassionate with yourself and focus on the progress you've made rather than dwelling on perceived mistakes. Consistency, not perfection, is the key to success.

Embracing Lifelong Prevention

Health is a lifelong commitment, and disease prevention doesn't end once you've achieved a certain goal or overcome a health scare. It's a continuous process of learning, adapting, and improving. The knowledge you've gained from this book should empower you to make informed decisions about your lifestyle and well-being, but your journey doesn't stop here.

1. Prioritize Health as a Lifestyle, Not a Phase

Prevention is best viewed as an ongoing lifestyle rather than a temporary phase. Embrace habits that nourish your body, mind, and spirit every day. Whether it's maintaining a balanced diet, staying active, managing stress, or nurturing your relationships, all aspects of your life play a role in keeping you healthy. By making these practices part of your routine, you create a sustainable approach to health that can support you for years to come.

2. Keep Educating Yourself

Health and wellness are constantly evolving fields, and staying informed will help you make the best decisions for your future. Continue to educate yourself about new research, techniques, and strategies for disease prevention. Books, articles, podcasts, and health seminars are all excellent resources for staying up to date with the latest information.

3. Adapt to Life's Changes

As you age, your health needs and risks may change. Embrace the idea that disease prevention strategies may evolve over time as you learn more about your body and experience new life stages. Be open to adjusting your approach, whether it's by incorporating new preventive screenings, revisiting your fitness regimen, or exploring different dietary approaches. The key is to remain flexible and adaptable, adjusting as necessary to optimize your health at every age.

4. Inspire Others

By embracing lifelong prevention, you set an example for others, especially those closest to you. Share the knowledge and practices you've learned with your family, friends, and community. Whether it's encouraging healthy eating habits, exercising together, or discussing mental health strategies, you have the power to inspire and positively influence those around you.

Appendices

Resources for Further Learning

1. Websites and Online Resources

° Centers for Disease Control and Prevention (CDC): www.cdc.gov
The CDC offers comprehensive guides on disease prevention, vaccinations, healthy living, and the latest public health data.

° World Health Organization (WHO): www.who.int
A global leader in public health, WHO provides resources on international health standards, disease prevention strategies, and wellness tips.

° National Institutes of Health (NIH): www.nih.gov
The NIH offers detailed information on various diseases, preventive research, and health programs, particularly for those seeking scientific-backed strategies.

○   American   Heart   Association   (AHA):
www.heart.org
For heart disease prevention, the AHA provides
resources   on   maintaining   cardiovascular
health, managing risk factors, and adopting
heart-healthy lifestyles.

2. Health and Wellness Apps

- **MyFitnessPal**: This app helps track
  your diet and exercise, making it easier
  to maintain a healthy lifestyle and
  prevent diseases related to poor
  nutrition and inactivity.

- **Headspace**: An excellent app for stress
  management and mindfulness, which is
  crucial for disease prevention.

- **Sleep Cycle:** Track your sleep patterns
  and gain insights into how to improve
  your sleep quality for better overall
  health.

3. Support Groups and Communities

º American Cancer Society Community: Provides online forums and support groups for those focused on cancer prevention and health.

º National Diabetes Prevention Program (NDPP): A community resource for people interested in learning about how to prevent type 2 diabetes through lifestyle changes.

Disease Prevention Glossary

- **Chronic Disease:** Long-lasting conditions that can be controlled but not cured, such as heart disease, diabetes, and cancer.

- **Inflammation**: The body's immune response to injury or infection, which, if persistent, can contribute to various diseases.

- **Insulin Sensitivity**: The body's ability to efficiently use insulin to lower blood sugar levels. High sensitivity is associated with better health outcomes.

- **Antioxidants**: Compounds found in foods that protect cells from damage by neutralizing free radicals, which contribute to aging and disease.

- **Microbiome**: The community of microorganisms living in and on our bodies, particularly in the gut, that influence our health and immunity.

- **Cardiovascular Health**: The condition of the heart and blood vessels, with good cardiovascular health being essential for preventing heart disease.

- **Mindfulness**: A mental practice that involves focusing on the present moment, reducing stress, and promoting mental well-being.

- **Prevention Strategies**: Actions and behaviors aimed at reducing the risk of developing diseases and improving long-term health outcomes.

Recipe Index

- **Superfood Smoothies**

- Green Antioxidant Smoothie:
  Kale, spinach, chia seeds,
  avocado, and almond milk

- Berry Detox Smoothie:
  Blueberries, flaxseeds, Greek
  yogurt, and lemon

- Tropical Turmeric Smoothie:
  Pineapple, coconut milk,
  turmeric, ginger, and a touch of
  honey

- **Anti-Inflammatory Dishes**

  - Salmon with Avocado Salsa:
    Omega-3 rich salmon served with
    an antioxidant-rich avocado salsa

  - Roasted Sweet Potato and Quinoa
    Bowl: A hearty bowl with sweet
    potatoes, quinoa, spinach, and a
    tahini dressing

  - Turmeric Chicken Stir Fry:
    Stir-fried chicken with turmeric,
    broccoli, and bell peppers

- **Heart-Healthy Meals**

  - Lentil and Chickpea Salad: A fiber-rich salad with lentils, chickpeas, cucumbers, tomatoes, and olive oil dressing

  - Grilled Vegetables with Olive Oil and Herbs: Zucchini, peppers, and mushrooms grilled with herbs for a low-fat side dish

  - Oatmeal with Almond Butter and Berries: A filling breakfast option to support heart health

- **Stress-Reducing Snacks**

  - Dark Chocolate and Almond Clusters: A sweet, antioxidant-rich snack to curb cravings while improving mood

  - Cucumber and Hummus Bites: A simple, crunchy snack packed with fiber and healthy fats

- Chia Pudding with Walnuts: A nutrient-dense snack that helps reduce inflammation and supports brain health

References and Recommended Reading

1. Books

° The China Study by T. Colin Campbell and Thomas M. Campbell II
A groundbreaking study on the relationship between diet and chronic disease prevention, particularly the role of plant-based diets.

° How Not to Die by Michael Greger, M.D.
This book explores the science behind preventing the top causes of death through diet and lifestyle changes.

° Why We Sleep by Matthew Walker, Ph.D.

An in-depth look at the importance of sleep for disease prevention and overall health.

2. Scientific Journals and Articles

° Journal of the American Medical Association (JAMA)
Regularly publishes research on disease prevention and health improvement strategies.

° The Lancet
A reputable medical journal covering global health, disease prevention, and lifestyle medicine.

° New England Journal of Medicine (NEJM)
Offers peer-reviewed research and reviews on the prevention of chronic diseases.

3. Websites for Continued Learning

° Harvard T.H. Chan School of Public Health
www.hsph.harvard.edu
Provides evidence-based research on nutrition, disease prevention, and public health topics.

° NutritionFacts.org

www.nutritionfacts.org A non-profit that offers free videos and articles on the latest health and nutrition research.

° Mayo Clinic
www.mayoclinic.org
A trusted resource for learning about diseases, prevention strategies, and healthy living.

By utilizing these resources, you can further deepen your knowledge of disease prevention strategies and continue your commitment to a healthier life.